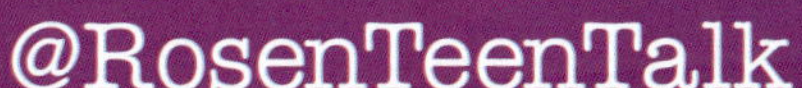

CANCER

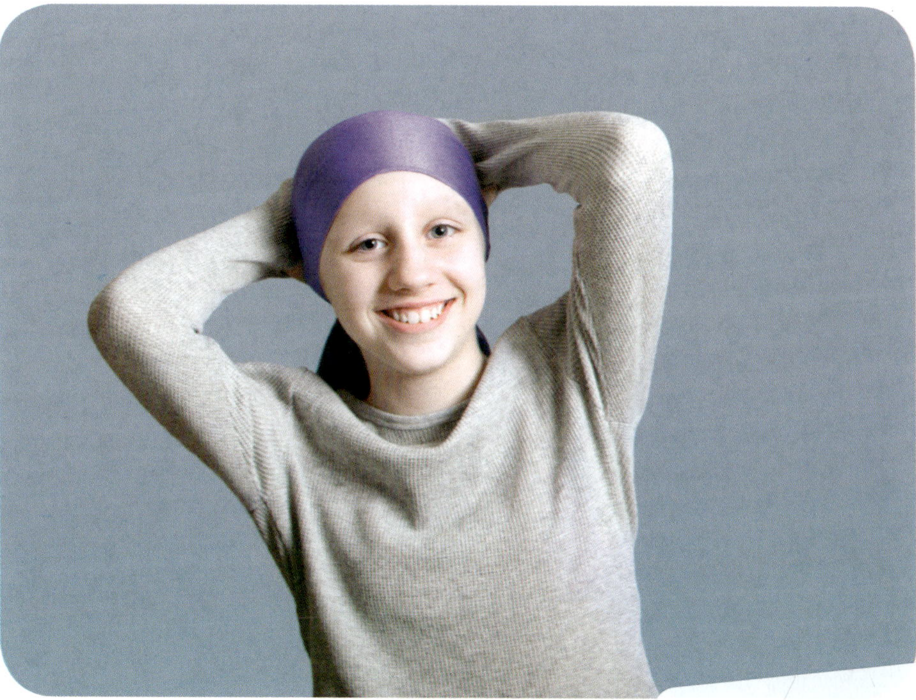

Corona Brezina

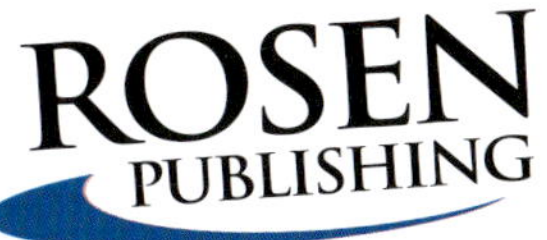

New York

Published in 2021 by The Rosen Publishing Group, Inc.
29 East 21st Street, New York, NY 10010

First Edition

Editor: Elizabeth Krajnik
Designer: Michael Flynn
Interior Layout: Rachel Rising

Photo Credits: Cover, p. 1 jessicaphoto/E+/Getty Images; cover Denis Gorelkin/Shutterstock.com; cover Cosmic_Design/Shutterstock.com; cover, pp. 1, 6, 8, 10, 12, 14, 16, 20, 22, 24, 28, 30, 32, 34, 38, 40, 42 Vitya_M/Shutterstock.com; pp. 3, 5 ©iStock.com/KatarzynaBialasiewicz; pp. 3, 19 Geber86/E+/Getty Images; pp. 3, 27 FatCamera/E+/Getty Images; pp. 3, 37 Image Point Fr/Shutterstock.com; pp. 3, 45 Maskot/Getty Images; p. 6, 38 Andrey_Popov/Shutterstock.com; p. 8 Ed Reschke/Stone/Getty Images; p. 9 Lisa F. Young/Shutterstock.com; p. 11 https://upload.wikimedia.org/wikipedia/commons/8/83/A_patient_is_prepared_for_radium_treatment_at_a_London_hospital_in_1940._D621.jpg; p. 12 James Leynse/Corbis Historical/Getty Images; p. 13 nobeastsofierce/Shutterstock.com; p. 15 Africa Studio/Shutterstock.com; p. 16 Morsa Images/DigitalVision/Getty Images; p. 17 New Africa/Shutterstock.com; p. 20 FG Trade/E+/Getty Images; p. 21 Simplylove/Shutterstock.com; p. 22 ER Productions Limited/DigitalVision/Getty Images; p. 23 TwilightShow/E+/Getty Images; p. 24 fluxfoto/E+/Getty Images; p. 25 Tyler Olson/Shutterstock.com; p. 29 Mark_Kostich/Shutterstock.com; p. 31 KARRASTOCK/Moment/Getty Images; p. 32 ARLOU_ANDREI/Shutterstock.com; p. 33 wavebreakmedia/Shutterstock.com; p. 34 Ariel Skelley/DigitalVision/Getty Images; p. 39 Den Rise/Shutterstock.com; p. 40 AshTproductions/Shutterstock.com; p. 42 Yulia Furman/Shutterstock.com; p. 43 Aleksandra Gigowska/Shutterstock.com.

Some of the images in this book illustrate individuals who are models. The depictions do not imply actual situations or events.

Library of Congress Cataloging-in-Publication Data

Names: Brezina, Corona, author.
Title: Cancer / Corona Brezina.
Description: New York : Rosen Publishing, [2021] | Series: @Rosenteentalk | Includes index.
Identifiers: LCCN 2020005237 | ISBN 97817499468045 (library binding) | ISBN 9781499468038 (paperback)
Subjects: LCSH: Cancer—Juvenile literature. | Cancer—Patients—Juvenile literature. | Cancer—Diagnosis—Juvenile literature. | Cancer—Treatment—Juvenile literature.
Classification: LCC RC264 .B74 2021 | DDC 616.99/4—dc23
LC record available at https://lccn.loc.gov/2020005237

Manufactured in the United States of America

CPSIA Compliance Information: Batch #BSR20. For further information contact Rosen Publishing, New York, New York at 1-800-237-9932.

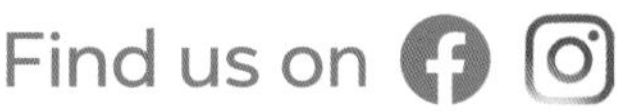

CONTENTS

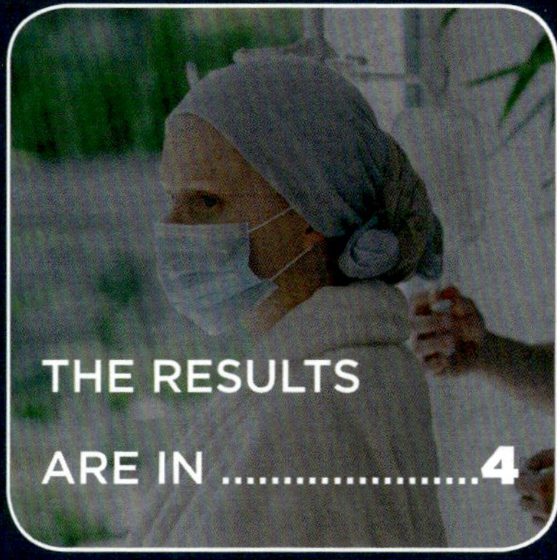
THE RESULTS ARE IN 4

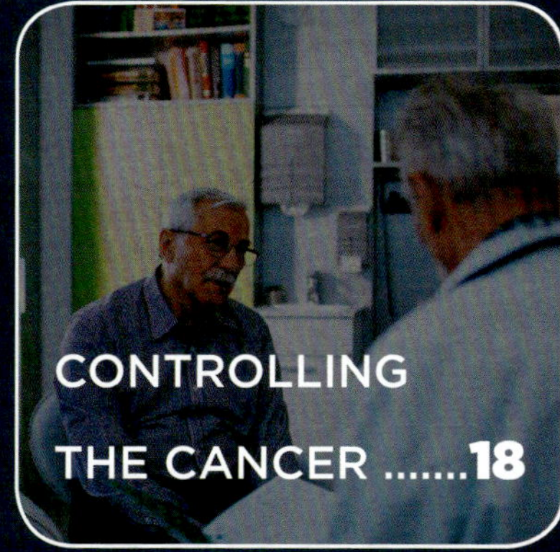
CONTROLLING THE CANCER 18

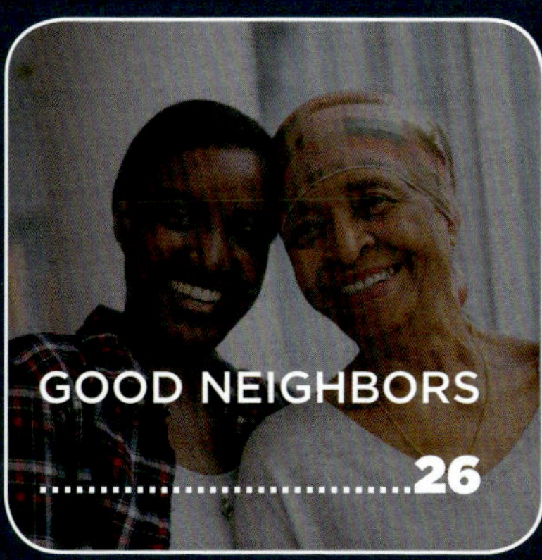
GOOD NEIGHBORS 26

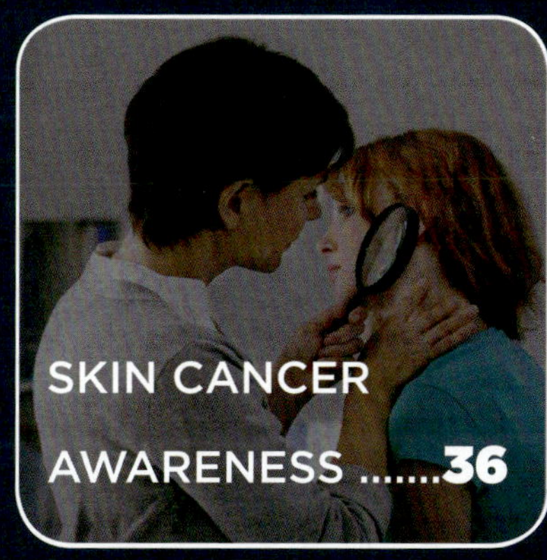
SKIN CANCER AWARENESS 36

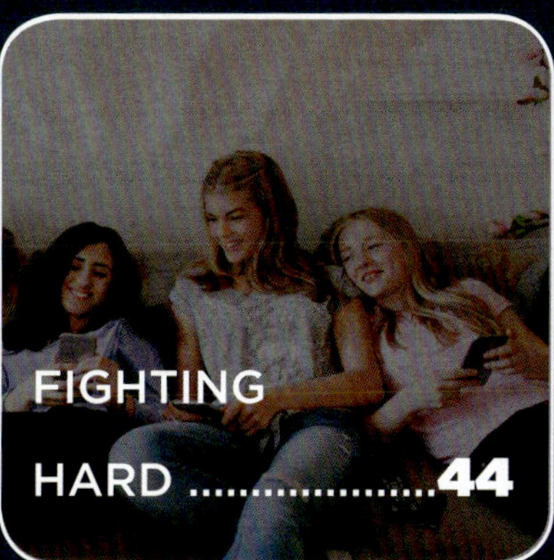
FIGHTING HARD 44

GLOSSARY 46

INDEX 48

Chapter 1

The Results Are In

Today I learned that I have cancer. It's called acute lymphocytic leukemia, or ALL. Leukemia is cancer of the blood.

I've been tired all the time lately. And I've had a fever. Sometimes, my **joints** hurt. I've been getting lots of **bruises** too.

My family doctor couldn't figure out what was wrong. So he ran a blood test. The results didn't look right. So he ran more tests. That's when he **diagnosed** me with ALL. He sent me to a doctor who specializes in treating childhood cancer. She and her team are going to help me get better.

ALL is a treatable form of cancer. But I'm scared about missing school. And I'm worried my friends won't understand what I'm going through.

Getting diagnosed with cancer is scary. But the more you know about it, the less scary it may be.

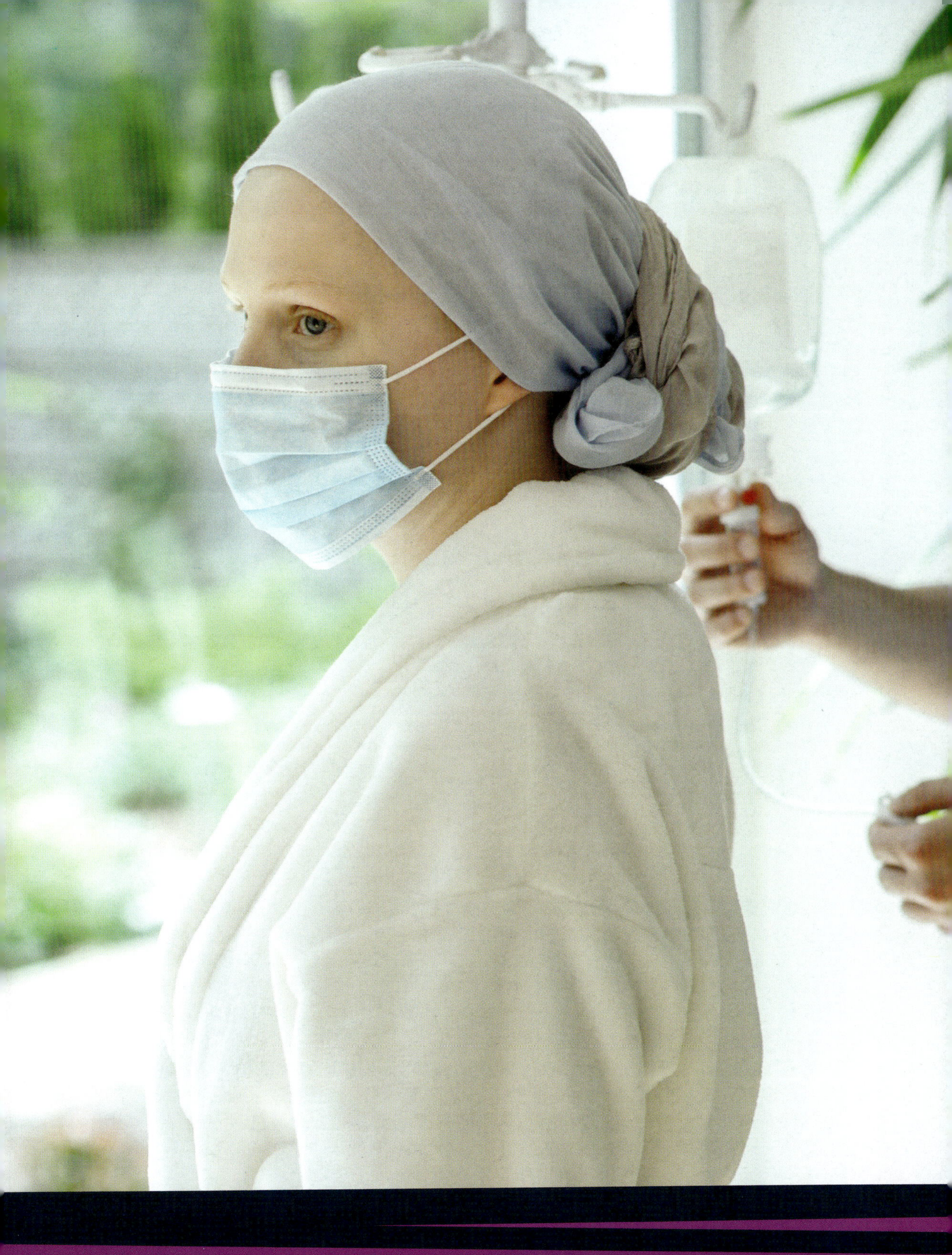

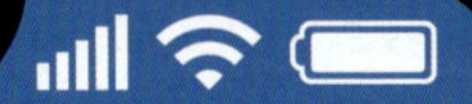

UNDERSTANDING CANCER

Cancer is a serious disease caused by **abnormal** cell growth. Cells are the building blocks that make up the human body. Cancer happens when cells grow out of control. If left untreated, cancer often spreads. It can harm **organs** and entire systems of the body. Cancer is the second leading cause of death worldwide.

Every year, more than 15,000 children and teens in the United States are diagnosed with cancer. Over 80 percent of young people with cancer survive.

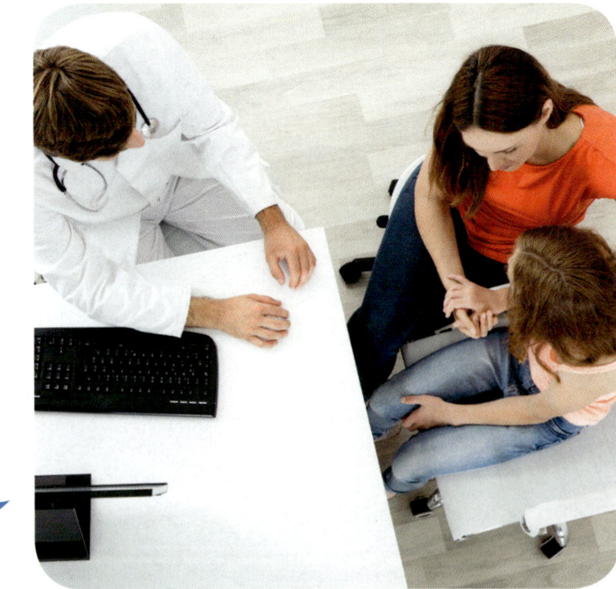

In the past, doctors couldn't do much to help people who had cancer. Today, many kinds of cancer can be successfully treated. **Researchers** are working to find new treatments.

Facts and Figures: U.S. Cancer Rates

About 1.7 million cases are diagnosed every year.

Each year, about 600,000 people die of cancer.

About 40 percent of people will develop cancer during their lifetime.

About 80 percent of all cases are diagnosed in people 55 and older.

FOR MORE INFORMATION

The American Cancer Society (**https://www.cancer.org/**) helps people learn more about cancer and treatments. The organization also conducts and funds, or puts money toward, cancer research.

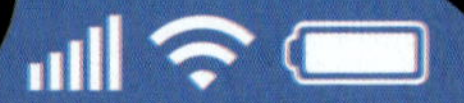

Normally, the cells in the body grow, split to form new cells, and then die. Cancer cells grow and split very quickly. Instead of dying, cancer cells survive and build up in the body. They may form **tumors**.

Cancer can occur in any part of the human body. Cancer isn't a single disease. There are more than 100 types of cancer. Some grow and spread more quickly than others. Different types of cancer respond better to different treatments.

The large purple cells in this blood sample are leukemia cells. There are a number of types of leukemia. Leukemias are the most common cancers in children. ALL is the most common type of leukemia in children.

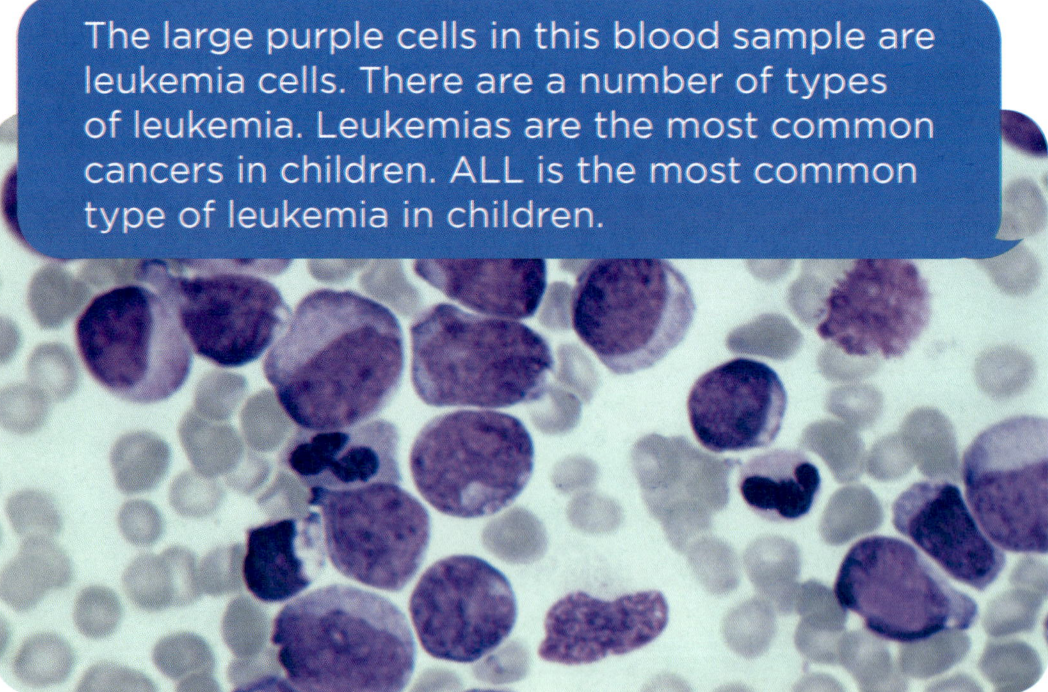

Meet the Doctor

Oncology is the branch of medicine that deals with preventing, diagnosing, treating, and studying cancer. A medical **professional** who practices oncology is an oncologist. An oncologist may specialize in studying or treating one type of cancer. Or they may do research.

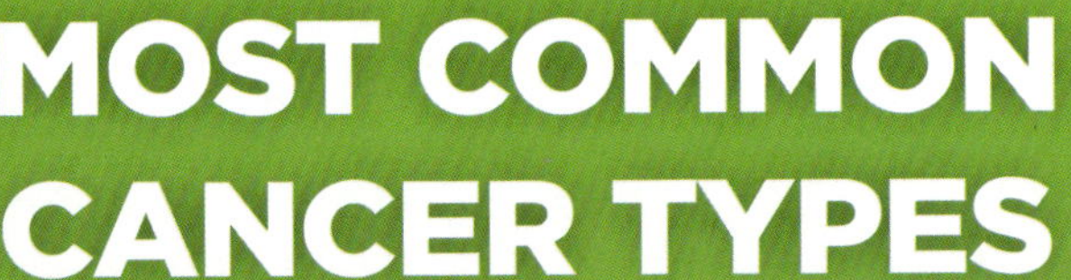

Some types of cancer are common. Other types of cancer are rarer. Here are some of the most common types of cancer and about how many new cases are diagnosed each year:

- Female breast (268,600)
- Prostate (174,650)
- Melanoma (96,480)
- Lung (228,150)
- Colon and rectum (145,600)
- Bladder (80,470)

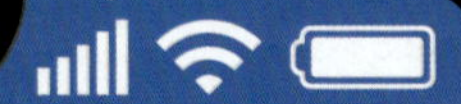

THE HISTORY OF CANCER

Cancer has affected humans throughout history. However, doctors only started to understand cancer in the 19th century. In 1882, William Halsted performed the first **surgery** to treat breast cancer.

In the 20th century, new **technology** made developing more effective treatments possible. In 1947, doctors began using drugs called antimetabolites. They stop cancer cells from splitting. Researchers began studying how cancer develops.

Today, there's still no cure for cancer. However, improvements in treatments mean many people survive.

In 1899, scientists began using **radiation** to treat cancer. It can kill cancer cells or keep them from splitting and spreading.

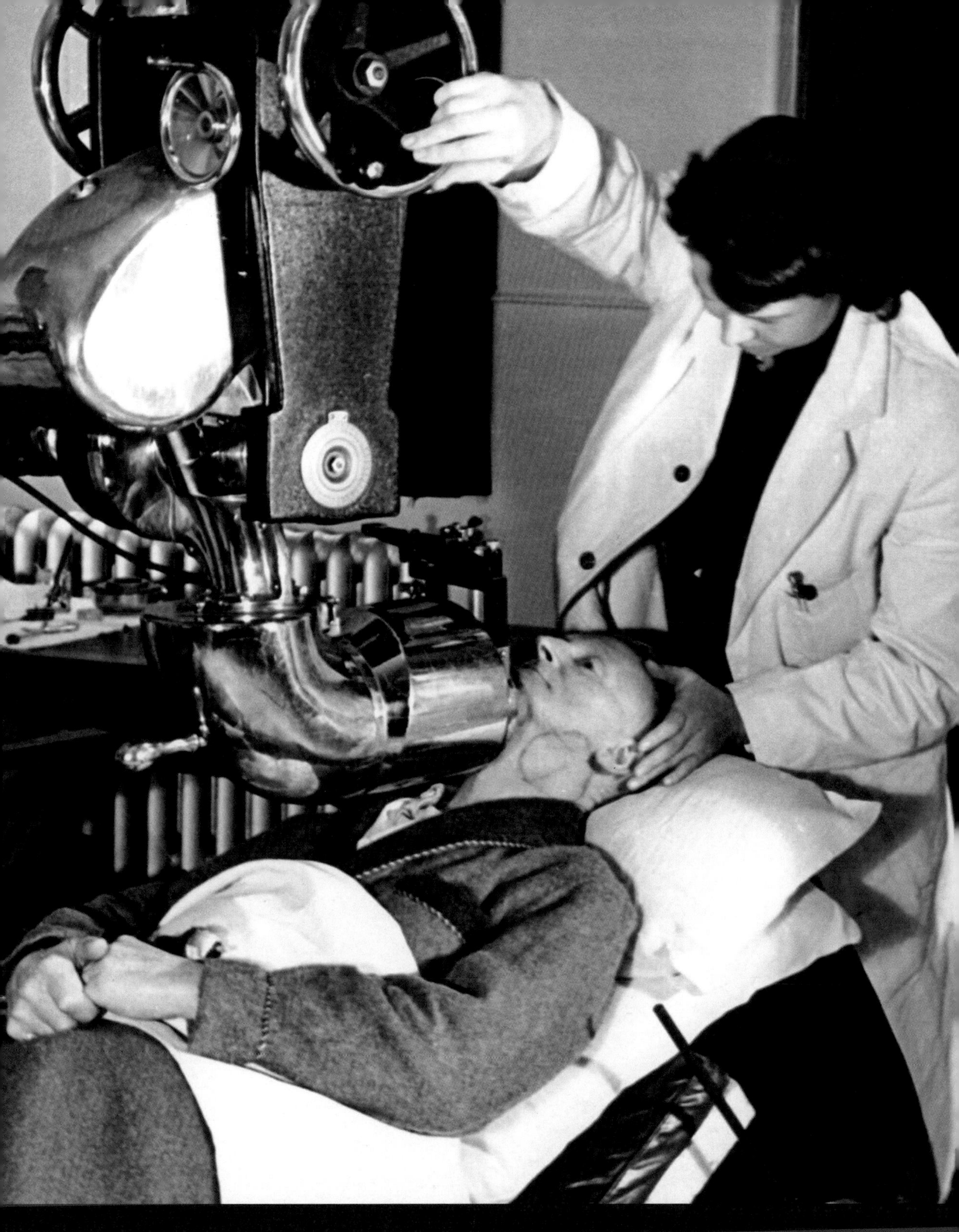

WHAT CAUSES CANCER?

In many cases, doctors can't find a single cause of someone's cancer. Most often, a number of causes have led to someone developing cancer.

Smoking tobacco products—such as cigarettes—can cause lung cancer and other types of cancer. Smokeless tobacco—such as chewing tobacco—can cause mouth cancer, other types of cancer, and other problems.

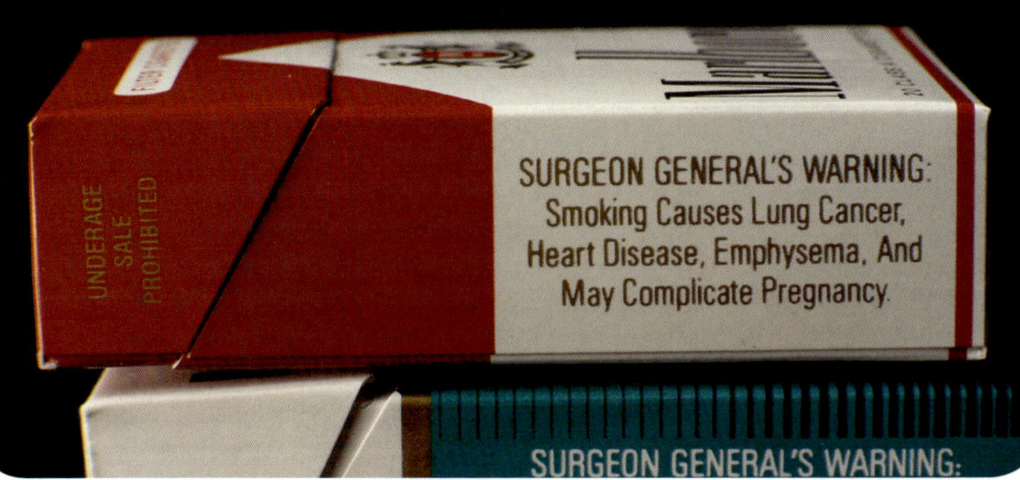

A risk factor is something that makes it more likely someone will develop a disease. Risk factors for cancer include someone's age, weight, the foods they eat, and how much they exercise.

Another risk factor for cancer is family history. About 5 to 10 percent of cancer cases are passed from a parent to children.

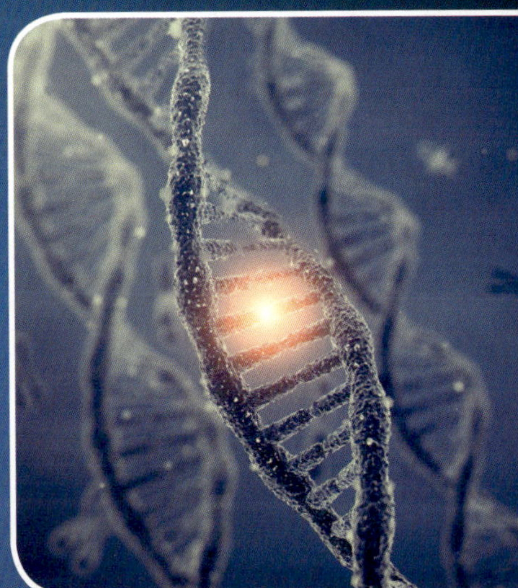

In the Genes

Doctors can run tests to see if someone has a higher risk of developing cancer due to certain **genetic mutations**. Young women who have mutated BRCA1 or BRCA2 genes are at greater risk of developing breast and ovarian cancer.

CARCINOGENS

Exposure to carcinogens is another risk factor for cancer. A carcinogen is a substance that can cause cancer. Here are some examples of known carcinogens:

- Tobacco
- Asbestos (building material)
- Alcohol
- Processed meat
- Air pollution
- UV rays (from sunlight or indoor tanning)

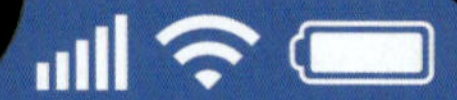

DETECTING CANCER

Cancer isn't always easy to **detect**. Someone may notice a change in their body. Or someone may be sick for a while and not get better. Their doctor may run tests to see if they have cancer.

COMMON CANCER SCREENING TESTS

TYPE OF TEST	TYPE OF CANCER	WHO SHOULD BE TESTED
Colonoscopy	Colorectal cancer	People between 50 and 75 years old
LDCT scan	Lung cancer	Heavy smokers between 55 and 74 years old
Mammogram	Breast cancer	Women between 40 and 74 years old
Pap test	Cervical cancer	Women between 21 and 65 years old

The earlier someone is diagnosed with cancer, the easier it is to treat. Early stages of cancer are less likely to spread. Doctors advise healthy people to be screened for certain types of cancer. People with a family history of cancer may undergo screening tests more often.

Performing a self-exam once a month can help people detect skin cancer early. If someone finds any areas of concern, they can show their doctor during a checkup.

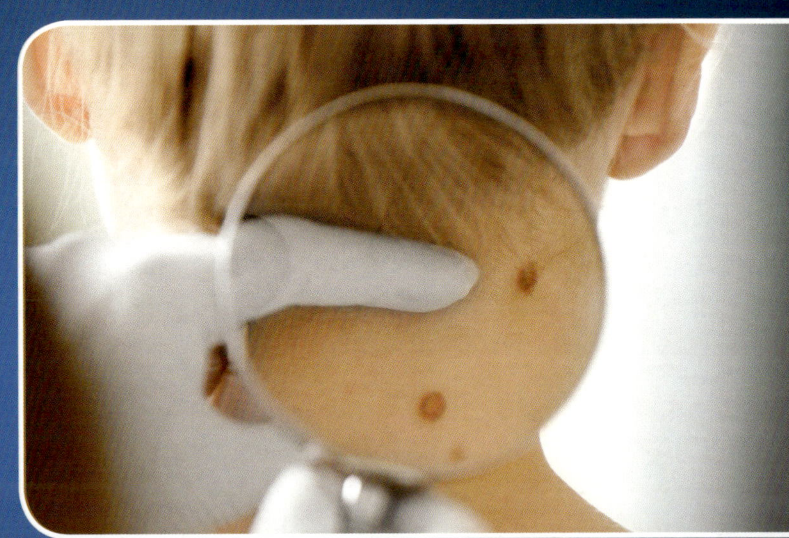

SYMPTOMS OF CANCER

Symptoms of cancer vary. Keep in mind, cancer isn't always painful. These are some common symptoms of cancer:

- Unexplained weight gain or loss
- Abnormal lumps or swelling
- Fever or night sweats
- Hoarseness or difficulty swallowing
- Fatigue
- Nausea
- Unexplained bleeding

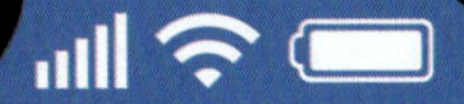

DIAGNOSING CANCER

Doctors use a number of different tests to diagnose cancer. Some cancers can be diagnosed from blood and urine tests.

Imaging tests produce pictures of the inside of a person's body. Doctors use the pictures to see if someone has a tumor and if cancer has spread.

Imaging tests show what's going on inside a person's body. They're usually painless. Doctors may perform imaging tests in a doctor's office, an imaging center, or in a hospital.

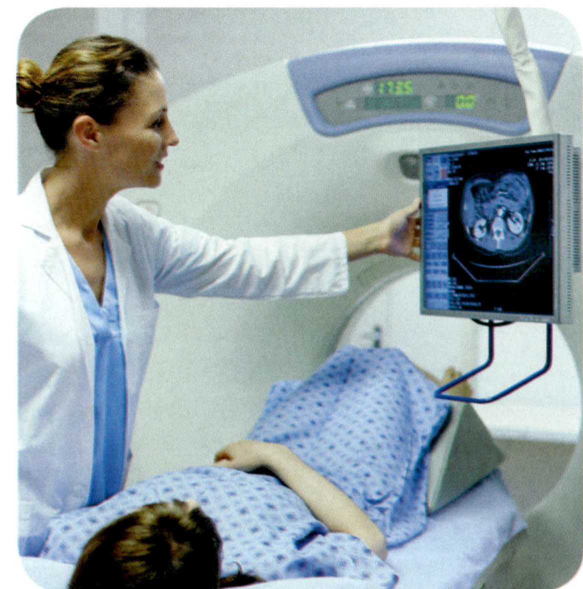

Cancer is most often diagnosed through a **biopsy**. Doctors examine the sample under a microscope to see if it's cancerous. They may also identify the type of cancer the person has.

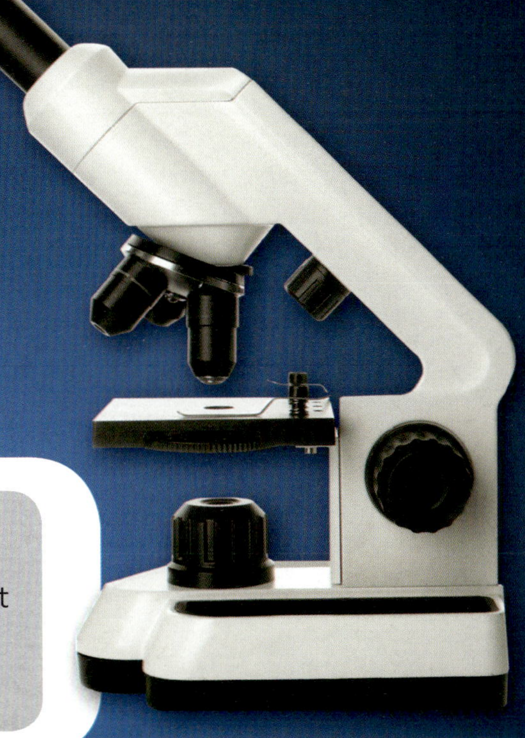

For More Information

Cancer.gov is the National Cancer Institute's website. The NCI is the government agency that carries out cancer research. The site provides **information** about cancer and different treatments.

TYPES OF IMAGING TESTS

- **X-rays:** Use radiation to show bones and organs
- **CT scan:** Uses precise X-rays to show bones, organs, and soft **tissues**
- **MRI:** Uses magnets to show soft tissues
- **Ultrasound:** Uses sound waves to show organs, soft tissues, and blood flow

Chapter 2

Controlling the Cancer

My grandfather is fighting prostate cancer. Prostate cancer grows very slowly. Grandpa isn't very strong. He has other health problems too. His doctors haven't yet decided which treatment is best for him. The treatment may cause more health problems than living with cancer.

Grandpa doesn't want to receive treatment. He'd rather his doctors treat the cancer symptoms. People can live with cancer for many months or years when their cancer is controlled.

I don't want Grandpa to suffer through painful treatments. But I'm scared that without treatment, he could die. My parents are having a tough time dealing with the news too.

We're all trying to learn as much as we can about Grandpa's type of cancer. Knowing what to expect helps us cope with his diagnosis.

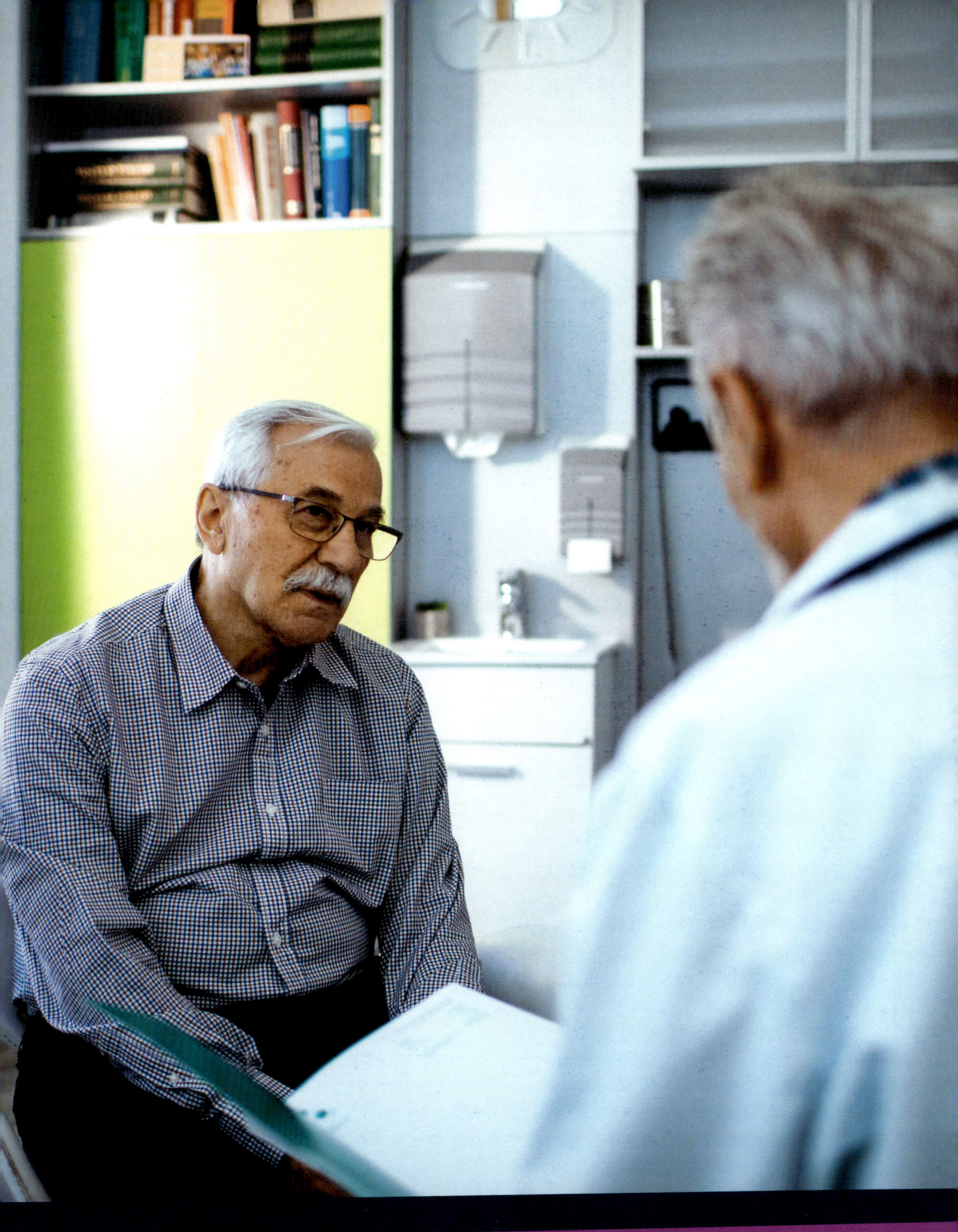

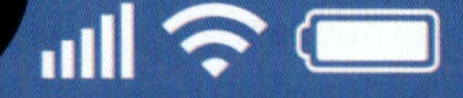

CANCER TREATMENT

Cancer is a **unique** disease. A treatment that works for one person may not work for another person. The treatment a person receives depends on a number of factors, including:

- Type of cancer
- Location of cancer
- Cancer stage
- Age
- Overall health
- How the person responds to treatment

Receiving cancer treatment has positive and negative effects. Some people choose the treatment most likely to cure their cancer. Other people choose the treatment with the least side effects.

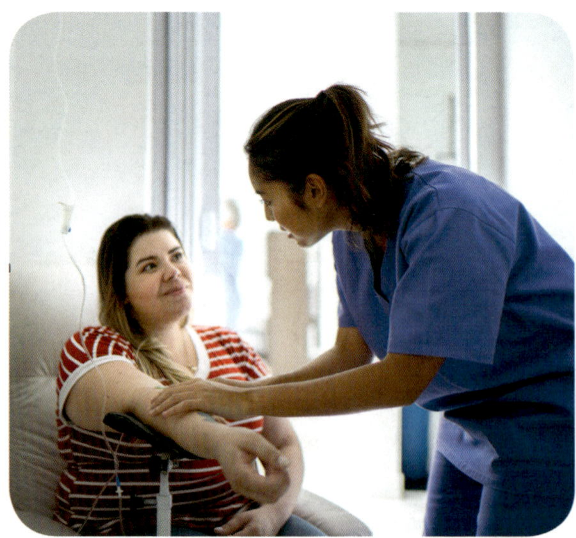

Often, the goal is to cure the person's cancer. Other times, the goal is to manage the cancer. Cancer treatments are hard on a person's body. People must take good care of themselves to stay strong.

Cancer Stages

Stage 0 No cancer is present.

Stage I Cancer is small and is present in a single spot.

Stage II and III Cancer is larger and has spread to nearby areas of the body.

Stage IV Cancer has spread to distant parts of the body.

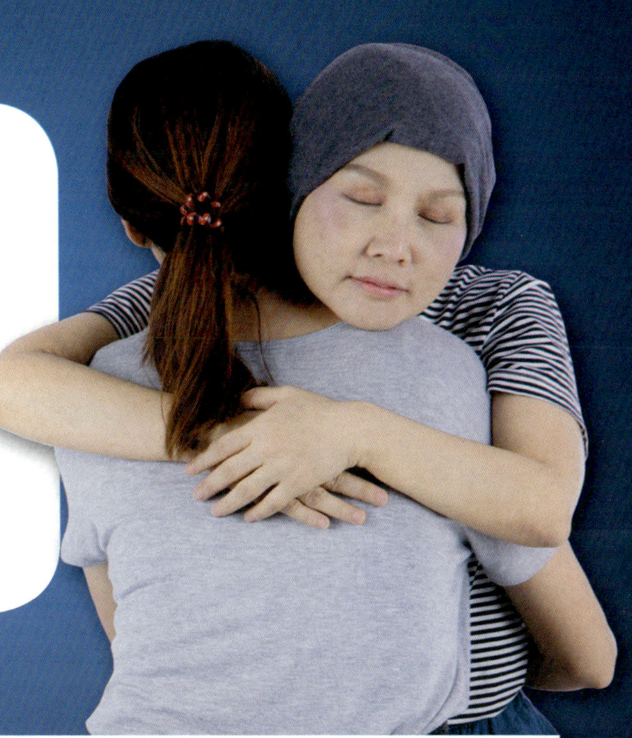

Emotional Self-Care During Cancer Treatment

- Share your thoughts and feelings with family and friends.
- Make time for fun activities.
- Join a cancer survivor support group.
- Talk to a **counselor** if you're feeling overwhelmed.

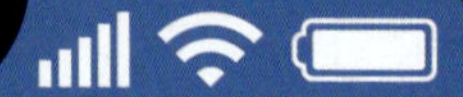

CANCER SURGERY

During cancer surgery, a doctor removes cancer from the body. A doctor who performs surgeries is called a surgeon. Surgery is the most common cancer treatment.

The surgeon may cut out a cancerous tumor. He or she may also remove tissue around the tumor. This is done to make sure that all of the cancer is gone.

Recovery times vary depending on the type of surgery. The person may have to take time off from work or school.

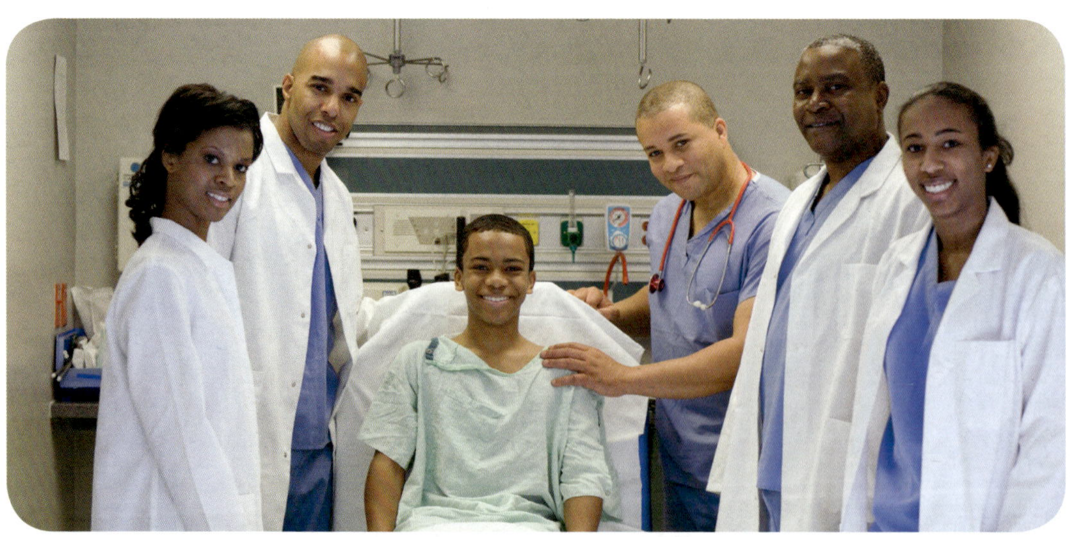

In some cases, people can go home right after their cancer surgery. In other cases, people have to spend time in the hospital.

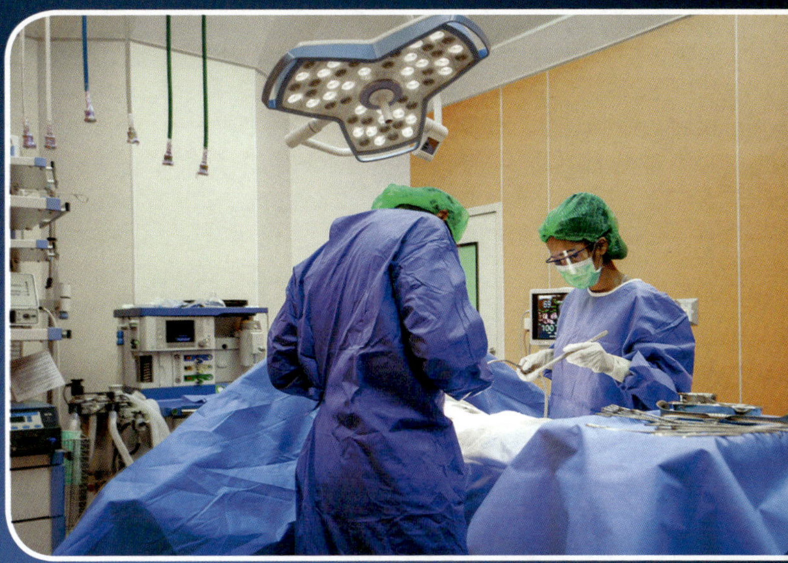

Reconstructive Surgery

Cancer and cancer treatment can change how the body looks. These effects are sometimes repaired with reconstructive surgery. For example, a woman may undergo a breast reconstruction after being treated for breast cancer.

TYPES OF CANCER SURGERY

- **Curative or primary:** Removes cancer from the body.
- **Debulking:** Removes some of the cancer when it's not safe to remove the entire tumor.
- **Palliative:** Treats problems related to advanced cancer, often to relieve pain.

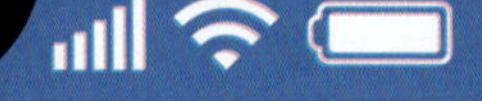

CHEMOTHERAPY

Chemotherapy is the use of drugs to treat cancer. Chemotherapy drugs kill cancer cells. But they also damage normal cells.

Chemotherapy may be someone's only cancer treatment option. More often, it's used along with other treatments. For example, someone may have cancer surgery. Then he or she will have chemotherapy to kill any remaining cancer cells.

Often, chemotherapy is given in cycles. The doctor gives the drugs over a few days or weeks. Then there will be a break before the next cycle.

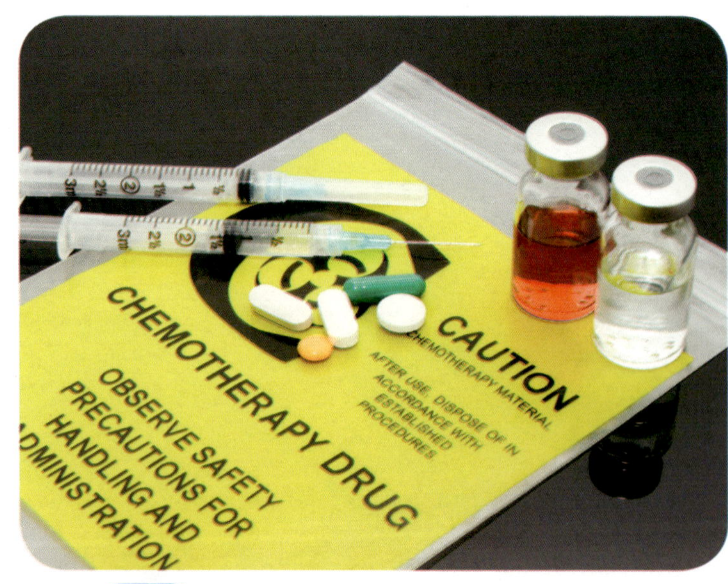

Teva's Story

In 2017, artist Teva Harrison was diagnosed with breast cancer. She described her battle with cancer in a graphic novel. It's called *In-Between Days: A Memoir About Living with Cancer*. The book tells the story of her diagnosis and treatment. She also talks about everyday life with family and friends as a person with cancer.

A doctor may treat someone with two or three chemotherapy drugs at the same time. Multiple drugs with different effects kill more cancer cells. This is called combination chemotherapy.

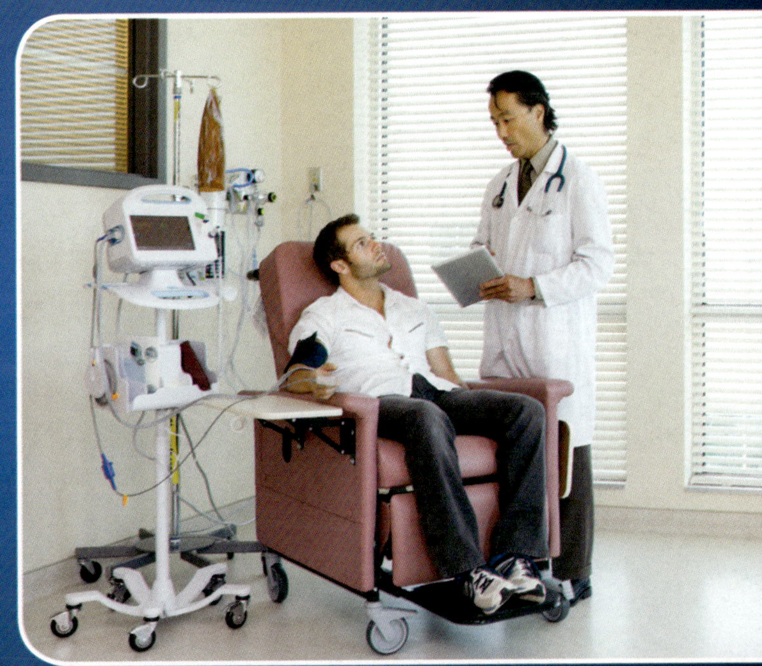

How Chemotherapy Is Given

- By injection (shot)
- Into a vein (IV)
- By mouth, as a pill or liquid

Chapter 3

Good Neighbors

Mrs. Lewis, my next-door neighbor, has breast cancer. She's had a lot of treatments so far—surgery, chemotherapy, and radiation. Mrs. Lewis has always been a great friend of our family. We're doing as much as we can to help her.

Mrs. Lewis can still keep up much of her daily routine. But she often gets tired. Her daughter drives her to doctor's appointments. She also helps around the house.

Mrs. Lewis likes it when we visit. We sometimes run errands for her. My dad sometimes brings meals over to her house so she doesn't have to cook. I've been helping out with yard work. But we're careful to stay away if we're sick. Mrs. Lewis's **immune system** can't fight off illness while she's being treated.

Even though Mrs. Lewis has hard days, she still finds joy in the company of her friends and family.

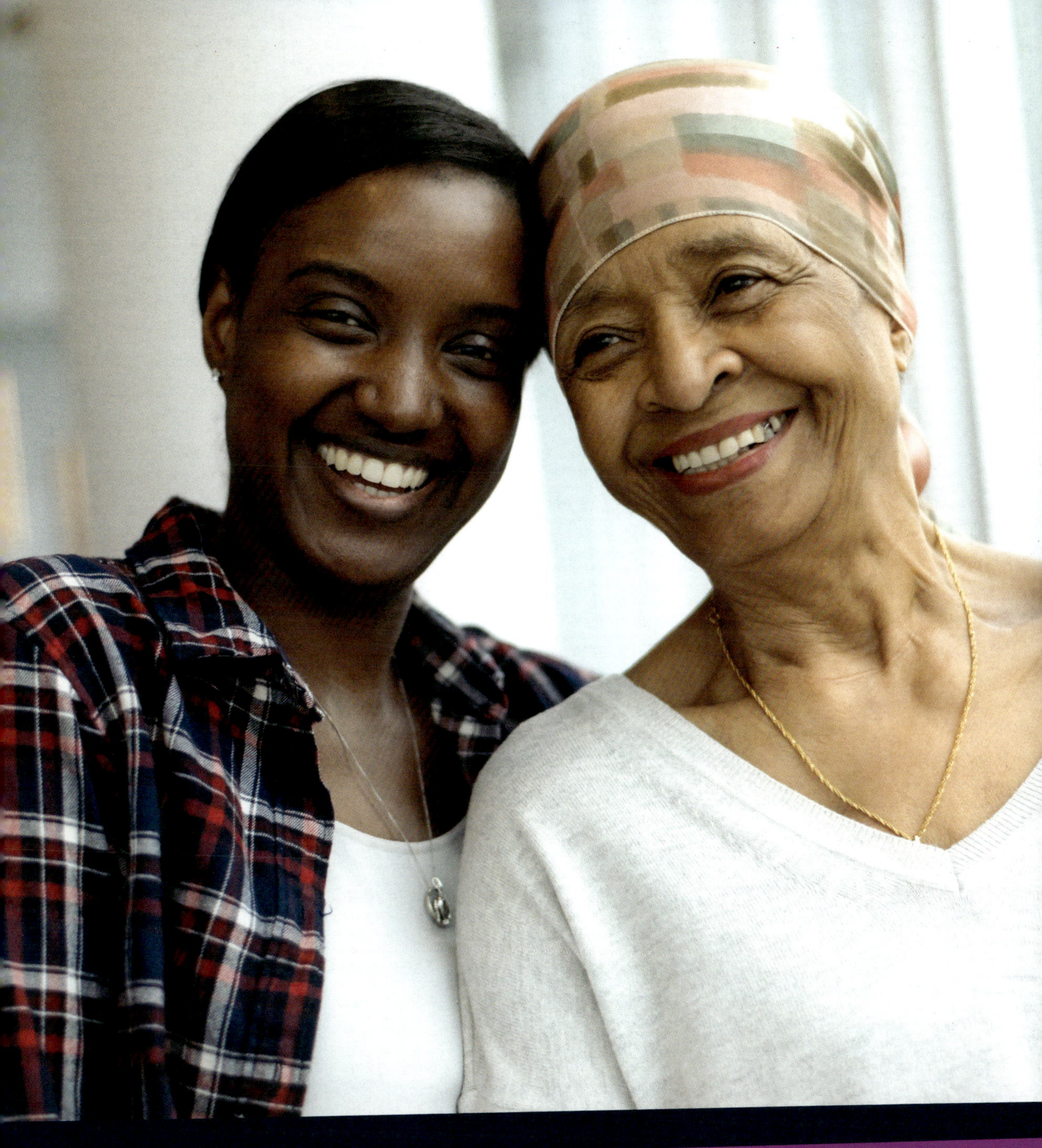

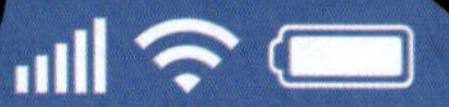

RADIATION THERAPY

Cancer patients may be treated with targeted radiation therapy. Radiation therapy uses X-rays or other high-energy beams. The machine targets the area of the body being treated. Radiation kills cancer cells. It makes tumors shrink. Nearby normal cells are also damaged.

Sometimes, a cancer patient is treated only with radiation. Or it can be combined with other treatments. Radiation can be given during cancer surgery. A patient treated with both radiation and chemotherapy may experience more side effects.

Radiation therapy is painless and only lasts for a few minutes. But people often feel tired after radiation treatments. People may experience painful side effects afterwards too.

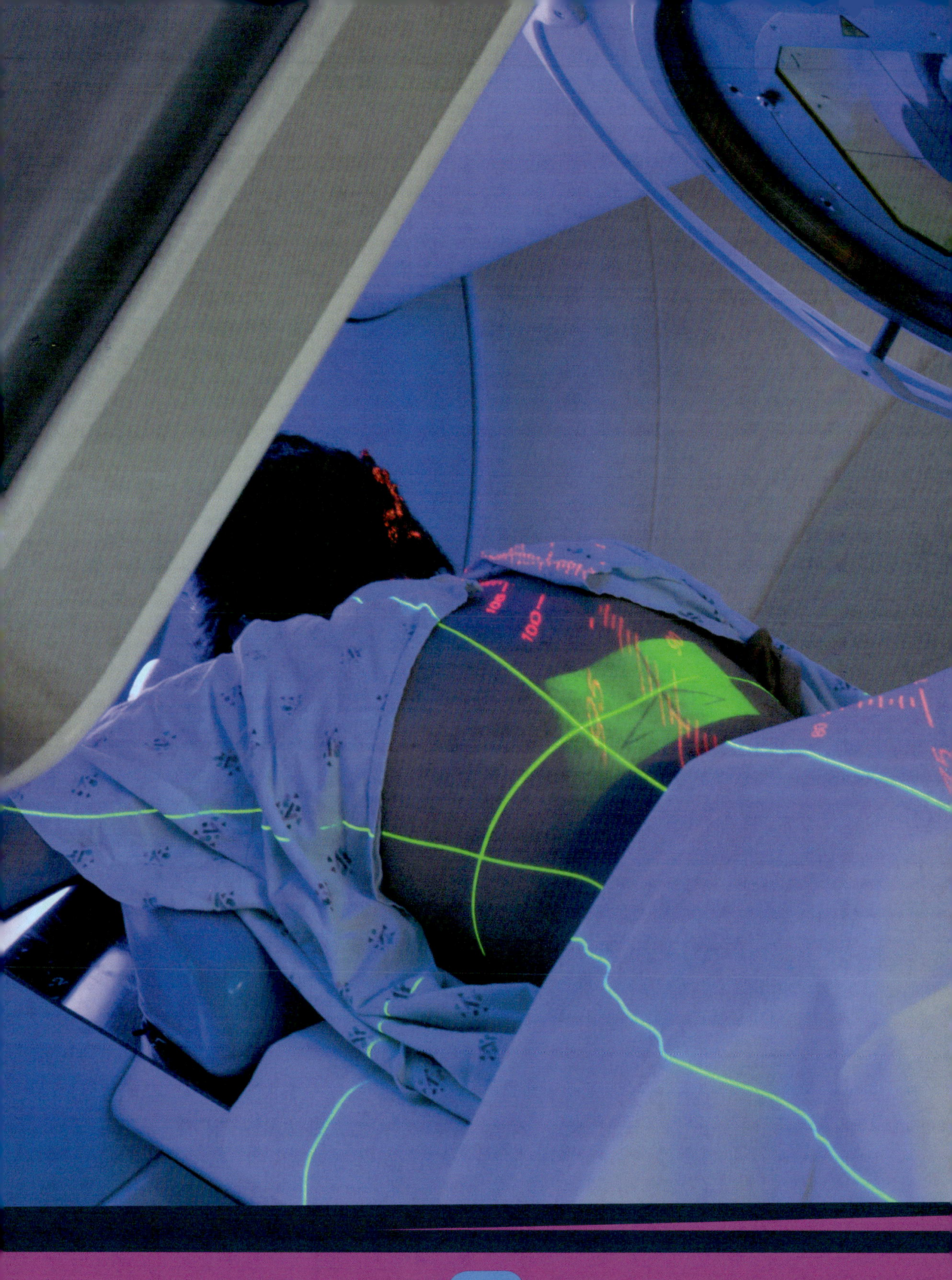

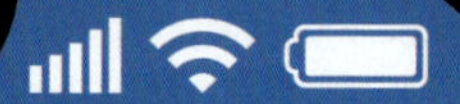

COPING WITH SIDE EFFECTS OF TREATMENT

Cancer treatments often cause severe side effects. People may feel very tired. They may also experience fevers, pain, and loss of appetite. People may have problems concentrating. They may also feel anxious or depressed.

Chemotherapy weakens the immune system. People undergoing chemotherapy treatments can get sick easily. Chemotherapy can also cause hair loss. Hair grows back after treatment.

Cancer treatments can also have long-term side effects. People who have been treated for cancer may have a higher risk for some medical conditions later in life.

Self-Care Questions for an Oncologist

How can I reduce the side effects of treatment?

What should I include in a healthy diet during treatment?

Can I exercise during treatment?

How can I deal with feelings of fear or anxiety?

Does the hospital offer survivor support groups?

Doctors encourage patients to maintain a positive attitude during cancer treatment. Patients should keep up their daily routines and fun activities as much as they can.

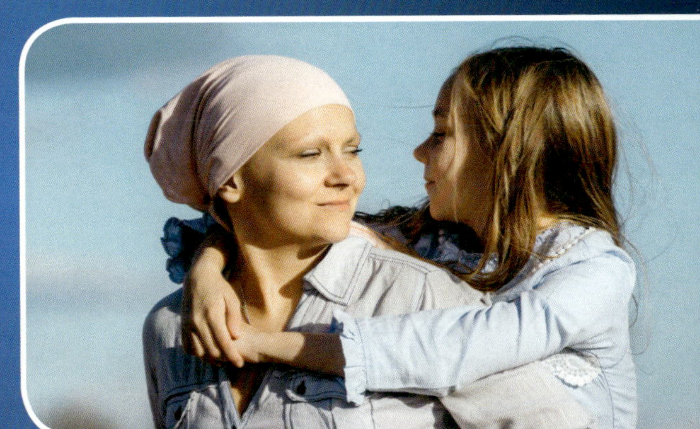

Possible Long-Term Side Effects of Cancer Treatment

- Bone loss
- Joint issues
- Hearing loss
- Eye problems
- Heart problems
- Lung problems
- Sexual health problems
- Fertility (having children) issues
- Tooth decay and other dental issues

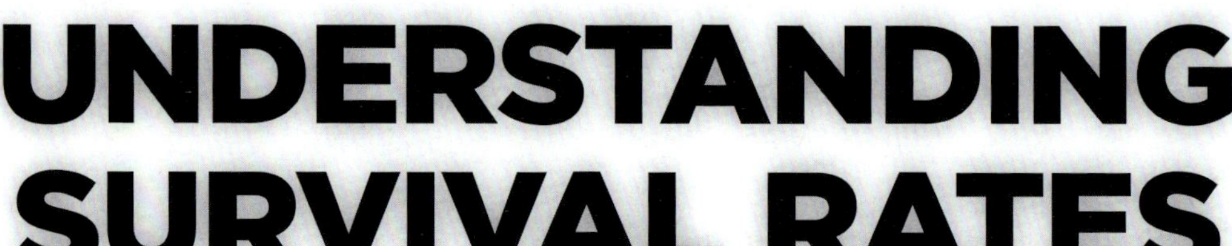

UNDERSTANDING SURVIVAL RATES

After a cancer diagnosis, the first question people often ask is, "Can it be cured?" Some forms of cancer respond better to treatment than others.

Doctors sometimes talk about survival rates. Survival rates describe the percentage of patients who survive cancer. Doctors often look at five-year survival rates. For example, the survival rate for breast cancer is 91 percent. That means that 91 percent of people treated for breast cancer are still alive five years later.

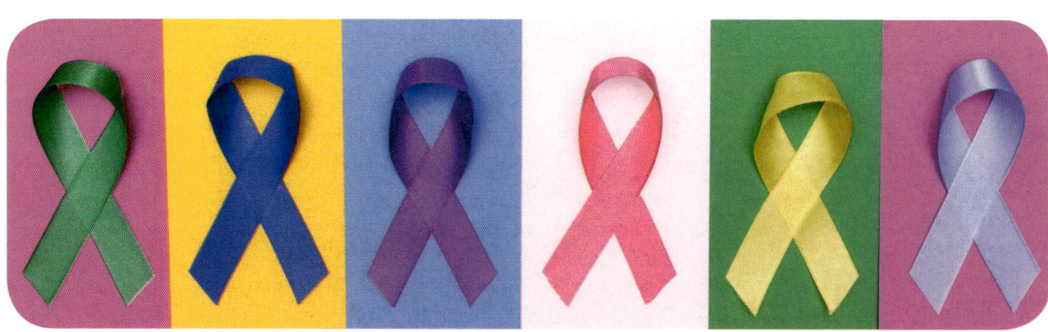

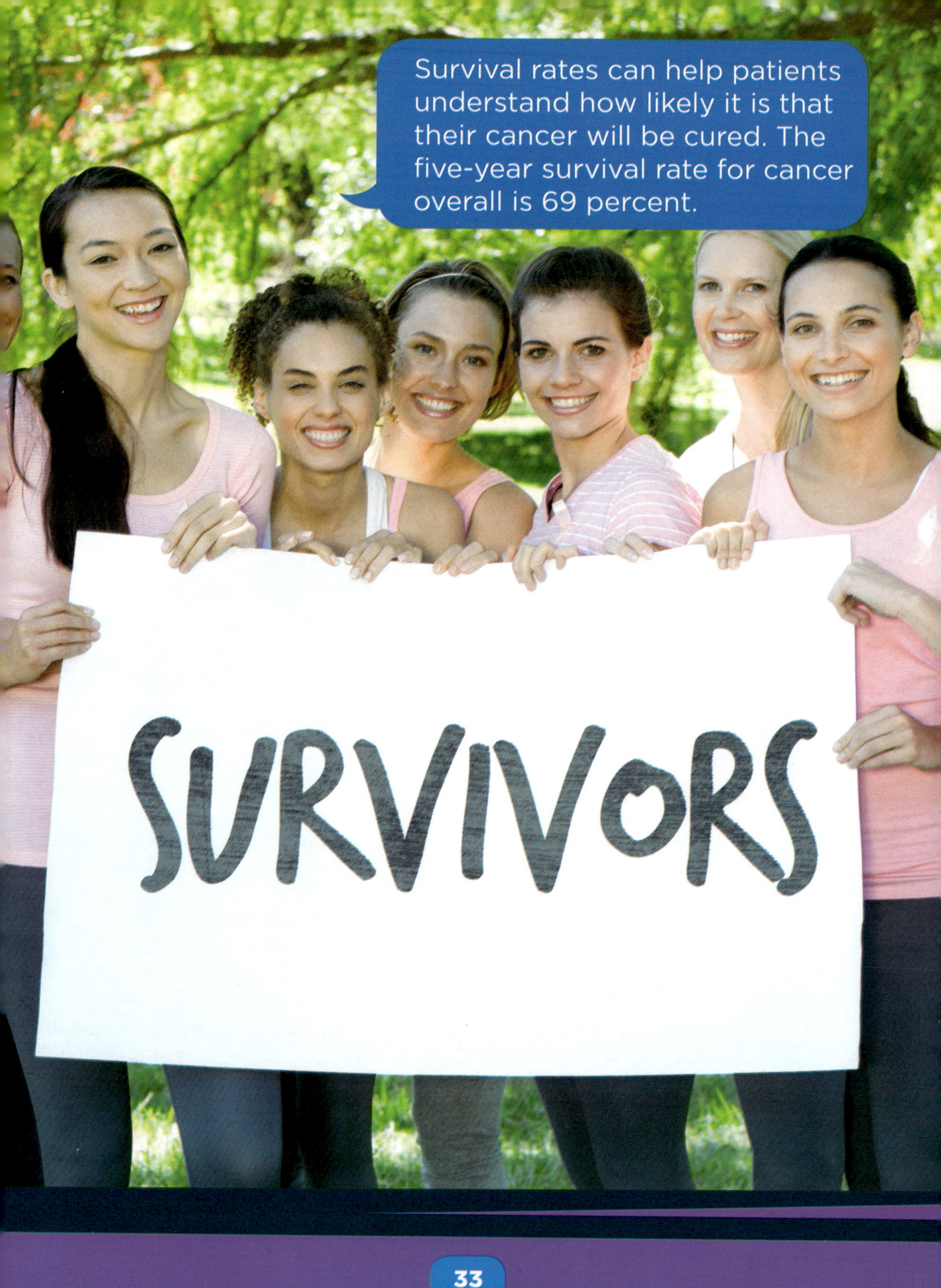

Survival rates can help patients understand how likely it is that their cancer will be cured. The five-year survival rate for cancer overall is 69 percent.

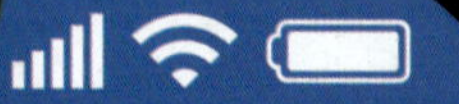

LIVING AS A CANCER SURVIVOR

After cancer treatment, patients return to their normal lives. But it takes time to heal. Some side effects take a long time to go away. Others may be permanent.

Often, the goal for cancer treatment is complete remission. This means that all signs and symptoms of cancer have disappeared.

Some cancer survivors practice **alternative medicine**, such as yoga, meditation, and massage therapy, to relieve pain or stress.

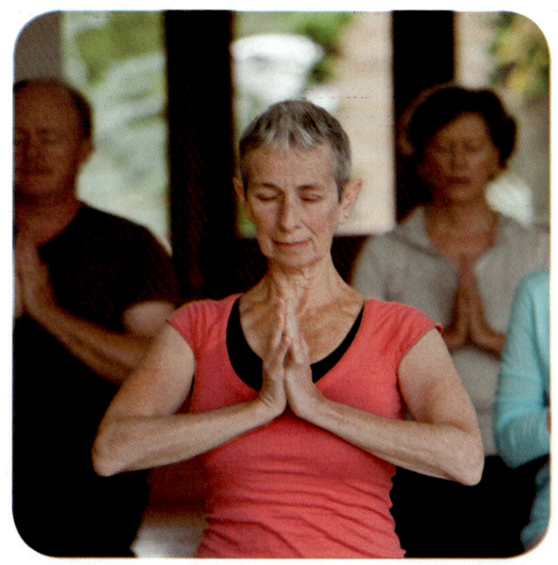

But cancer can recur, or come back. After a successful treatment, a survivor will continue to have follow-up visits. The doctor will check whether the cancer has recurred.

Resources for Survivors

Survivorship: Cancer.net
https://www.cancer.net/survivorship
This site provides readers with information about surviving cancer for cancer survivors and the people in their lives.

Children's Oncology Group
http://www.survivorshipguidelines.org/
This website has detailed long-term follow-up guidelines for young cancer survivors.

Cancer Center – Nemours KidsHealth
https://kidshealth.org/en/teens/center/cancer-center.html?ref=search
This website has a wealth of information about cancer for teens, including how to deal with cancer.

CANCER AND FERTILITY

Cancer treatment can make it harder for survivors to have children. Sometimes, they freeze their sperm or eggs before undergoing cancer treatment. Others may undergo fertility treatments later on to help them start a family. Or they may choose to adopt.

Chapter 4

Skin Cancer Awareness

Last year I had my yearly checkup. My doctor was worried about a mole on my skin. He took a sample for testing. It turned out that I had skin cancer. I couldn't believe it.

The cancer was easily removed through surgery. The treatment was successful. But I was lucky. Some cases of skin cancer can be very serious.

Since my treatment, I've been working to raise awareness about skin cancer. Cancer rates have been rising among teens. I should have been more careful about protecting my skin from the sun. Sunburns can be dangerous. Indoor tanning also raises skin cancer risk.

I've taught my friends how to recognize signs of skin cancer. It's important to catch it early.

A lot of my friends like to get tan in the summer. But I told them how dangerous it can be. Some of them have gone to the doctor to get their skin checked.

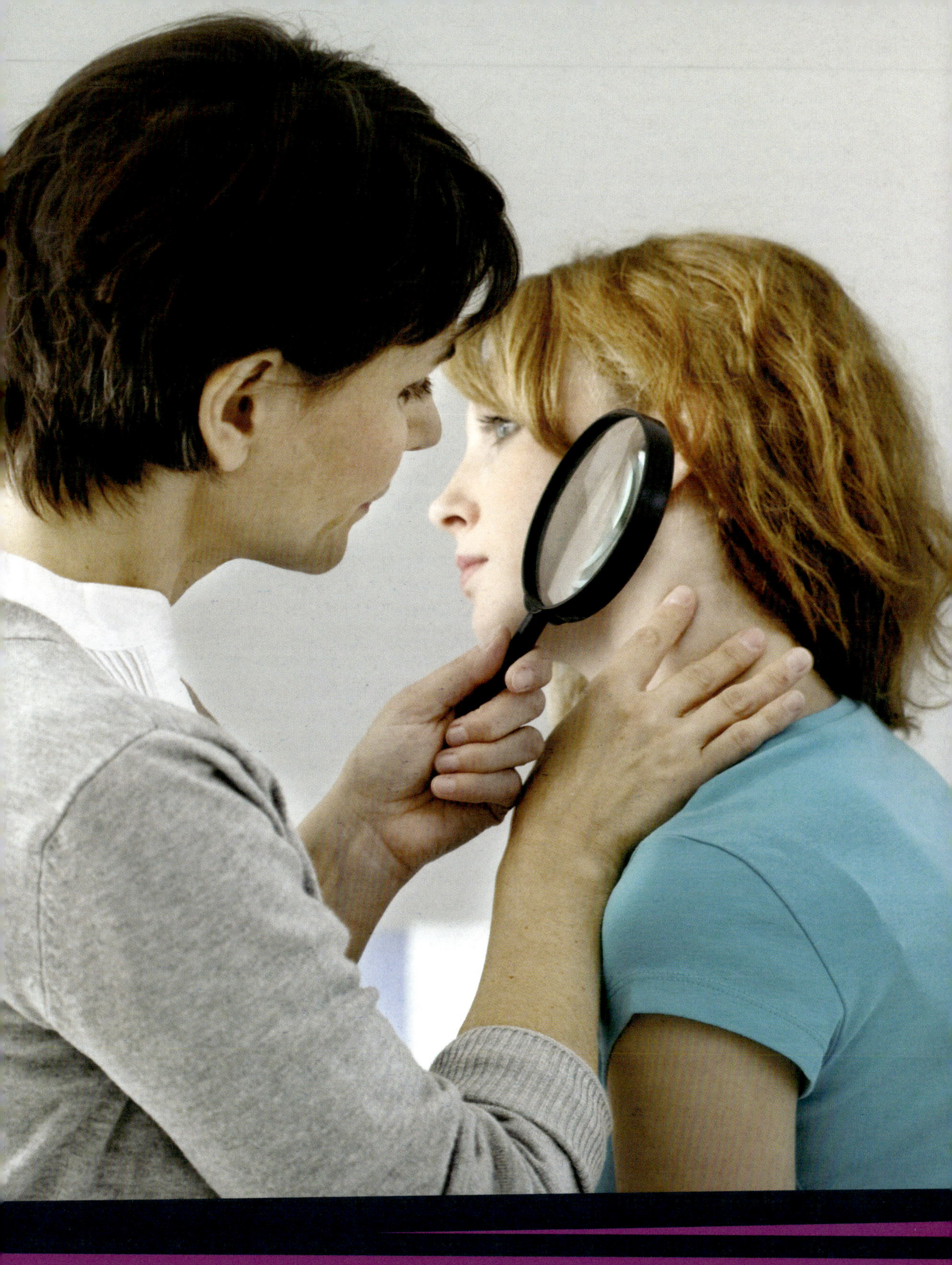

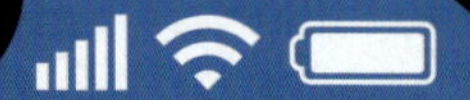

CANCER RECURRENCE

Every cancer patient fears that their cancer will come back. If some cancer cells aren't killed during treatment, cancer can return months or even years after remission. Some types of cancer are more likely to recur than others.

A doctor may diagnose someone with a cancer recurrence after routine tests. The person may also show symptoms that are diagnosed as a recurrence.

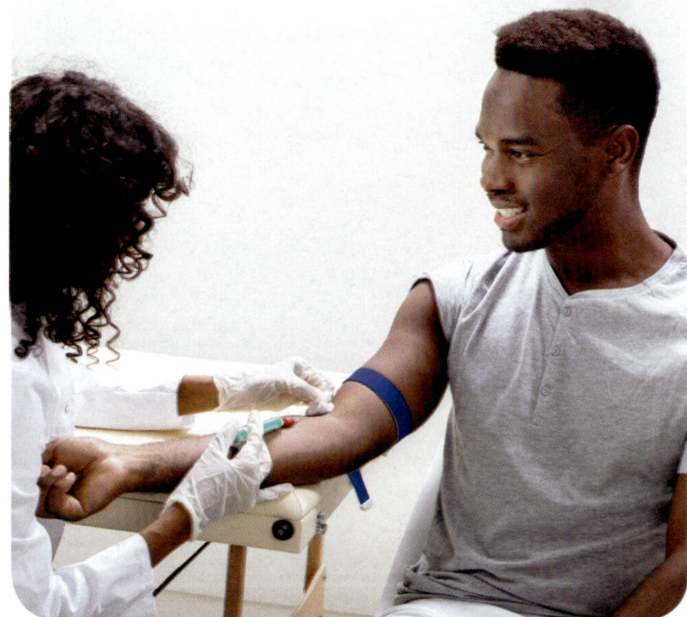

Cancer that recurs can be more difficult to treat. It may not respond as well to the original treatment method. Doctors may have to try a different type of treatment. Cancer that recurs is often treated successfully. It can also be controlled.

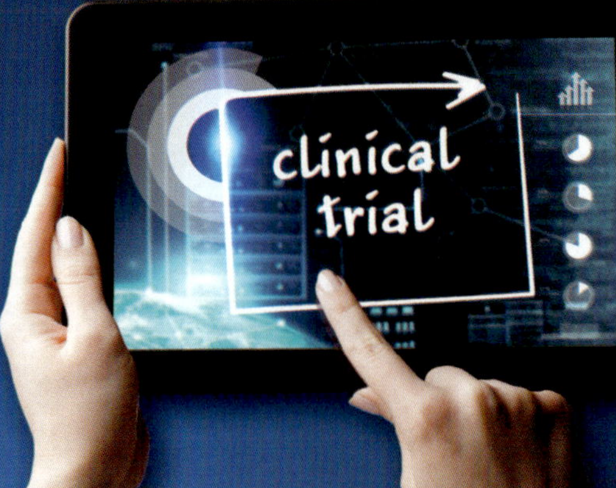

Clinical Trials

People who have cancer that has come back may choose to take part in a clinical trial. This is when a new type of treatment or medicine is tested on humans. Clinical trials aren't guaranteed to help people. But they may improve someone's chances of getting better.

TYPES OF RECURRENCE

- **Local recurrence:** The cancer returns in the same place.
- **Regional recurrence:** The cancer returns to a place nearby the original cancer.
- **Distant recurrence:** The cancer has spread to organs or tissues far from the original cancer.

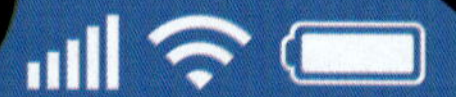

WORKING TOWARD A CURE

In 1971, President Richard Nixon signed the National Cancer Act. Some people believed the law would mean that researchers would quickly find a cure for cancer. Doctors and researchers still haven't found a cure for cancer. But cancer prevention, treatments, and survival rates have improved.

The first chemotherapy drugs were developed in the 1950s. Today, there are more than a hundred different chemotherapy drugs. Researchers continue to develop and test new drugs.

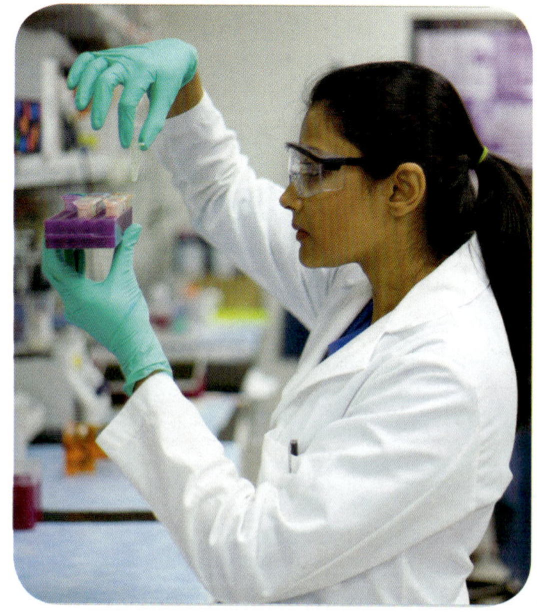

Scientists and doctors continue to conduct cancer research in hospitals and labs. They work to learn more about how cancer works. The more they understand, the better able they are to create new, more effective cancer treatments.

New Cancer Treatment: Immunotherapy

Immunotherapy uses the immune system to fight cancer. It has been successful in treating some types of cancer. Researchers hope that new immunotherapy drugs can help treat more types of cancer. Immunotherapy often has fewer side effects than other cancer treatments.

AREAS OF CANCER RESEARCH

- Cancer biology—how cancer works
- Diagnosis and screening
- Public health
- Clinical trials
- Causes of cancer
- Prevention
- Childhood cancer
- Treatments

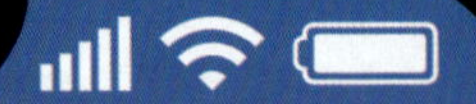

REDUCING YOUR RISK OF CANCER

Healthy lifestyle choices can reduce your risks of developing some types of cancer. Regular exercise and eating a balanced diet is a great start. Maintaining a healthy weight and protecting yourself from the sun helps reduce cancer risk too. You should also avoid using tobacco products.

Certain foods are known as cancer-fighting superfoods. They can also improve your overall health. If you eat plenty of these foods, you may stay healthier for longer.

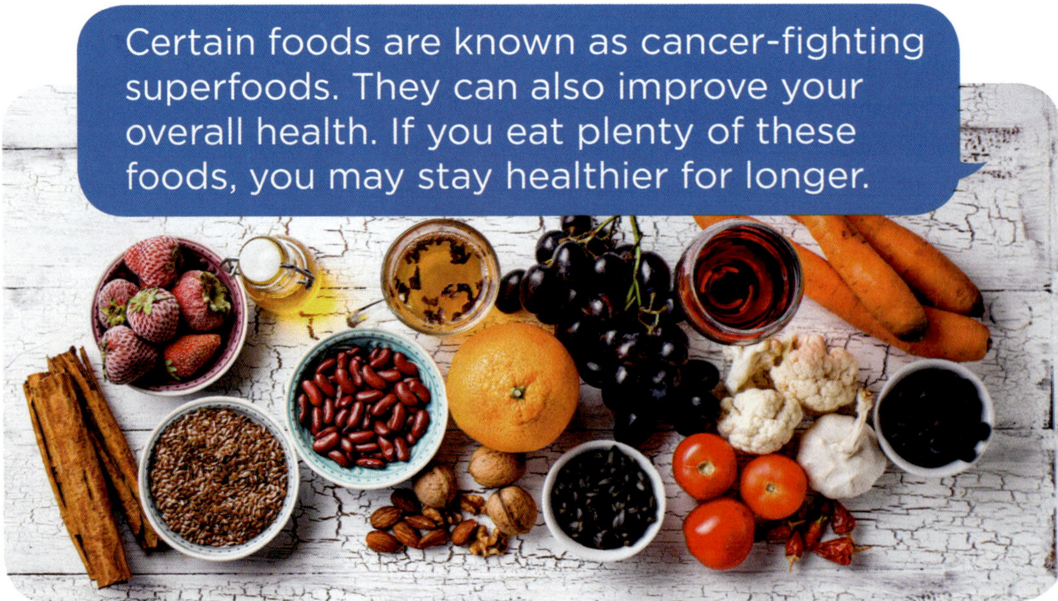

Vaccines can prevent some cancers. The **HPV** vaccine, for example, protects against the types of HPV that most often cause a number of cancer types in women. If you have a family history of cancer, you should get screened.

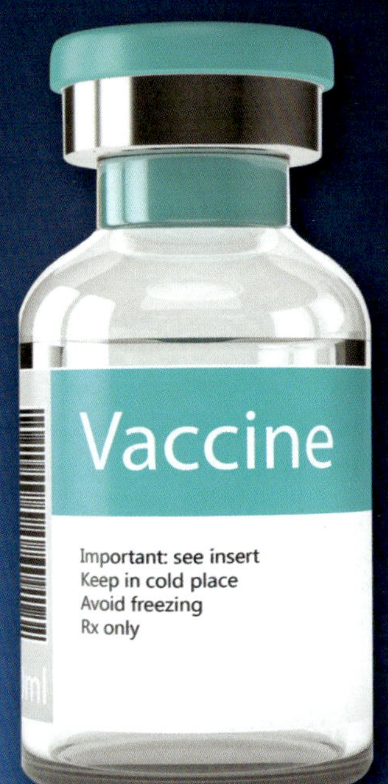

For More Information

The Anti-Cancer Diet **by oncologist Dr. David Khayat**
Learn how what you eat can reduce your cancer risk.

Office of Disease Prevention and Health Promotion
https://health.gov
Read about how healthy lifestyle choices can positively affect your overall health and wellness.

MAKE A DIFFERENCE

Stay in shape and raise money to fight cancer! Sign up for a fun run or other charity event. You can find out about events in your area by asking at your local hospital. Or check with organizations such as the American Cancer Society (**https://www.cancer.org/**).

Chapter 5

Fighting Hard

I had some good news today! My doctor told me the leukemia cell count in my blood has dropped a lot. This means my cancer is responding well to treatment!

I've been having chemotherapy treatments for about two months now. My oncologist started treatment as quickly as she could. That's because the cancer grows so fast. The first month was the worst. I was on several different chemotherapy drugs. I had to stay in the hospital.

I'm going to have to continue chemotherapy for about two years. Over time, I'll get less of the chemotherapy drugs. The chemotherapy should kill all the cancer cells.

My friends have been great. Chemotherapy made my hair fall out. They helped me pick out a wig that looks like my real hair!

My friends make time to see me even if I miss school. They're happy to sit with me and watch movies if I'm too tired.

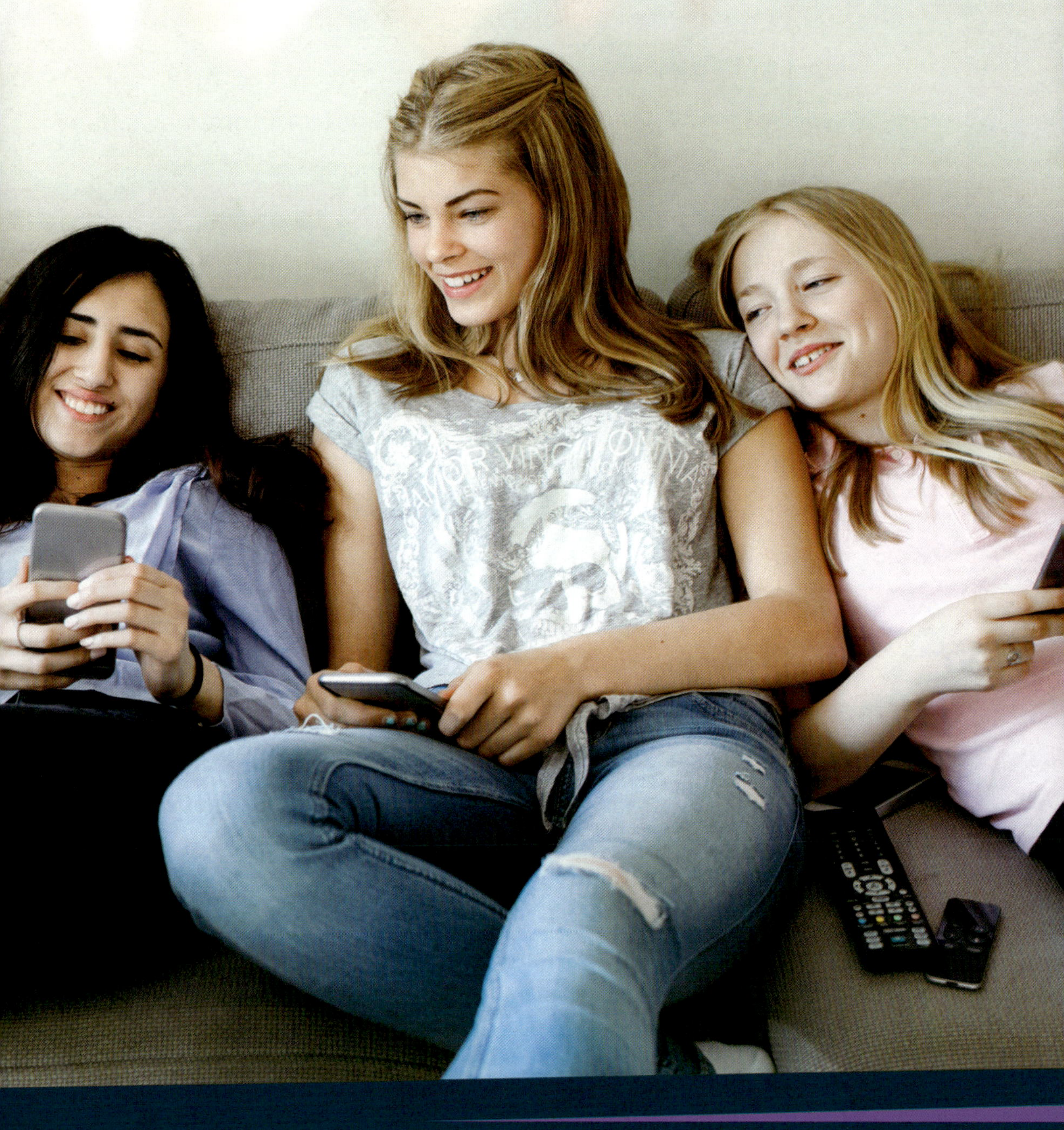

GLOSSARY

abnormal: Differing from the normal usually in a noticeable way.

alternative medicine: Any way of healing or treating disease that differs from Western medicine.

biopsy: The removal of tissue, cells, or fluids from someone's body in order to check for illness.

bruise: A dark and painful area on a person's skin that is caused by an injury.

counselor: A person who provides advice as part of their job.

detect: To learn that something or someone is or was there.

diagnose: To identify a disease by its signs and symptoms.

genetic mutation: A mistake or change in a living thing's DNA that causes the living thing to have a different trait.

HPV: Human papillomavirus. A virus that infects the skin, genital area, and lining of the cervix. It is spread during unprotected sex with an infected partner.

immune system: The system that protects the body from diseases and infections.

information: Knowledge or facts about something.

joint: A point where two bones meet in the body.

organ: A body part that does a certain task.

professional: A person who does a job that requires special education or skill.

radiation: The use of controlled amounts of radiation, or energy that comes as waves or rays you can't see, for the treatment of diseases.

researcher: Someone who does research, or careful study to find new knowledge.

surgery: Medical treatment in which a doctor cuts into someone's body in order to repair or remove damaged or diseased parts.

symptom: A sign that someone is sick.

technology: A method that uses science to solve problems and the tools used to solve those problems.

tissue: A group of cells of the same kind that come together to form the basic parts that make up a plant or animal.

tumor: An abnormal growth of body tissue.

unique: Special or different from anything else.

vaccine: A substance that is usually injected into a person or animal to protect against a particular disease.

INDEX

B
biopsy, 17
breast cancer, 9, 10, 13, 14, 23, 25, 26, 32
bruises, 4

C
carcinogens, 13
cells, 6, 8, 10, 24, 28, 38, 44
chemotherapy, 24, 25, 26, 28, 30, 44
clinical trials, 39, 41
counselor, 21
cure, 10, 21, 32, 40

D
diagnosis, 4, 7, 9, 15, 16, 17, 18, 25, 32, 41
doctors, 4, 7, 9, 10, 12, 13, 14, 15, 16, 17, 18, 22, 24, 26, 32, 35, 36, 39, 40, 41, 44

F
family history, 13, 15
fever, 4, 15, 30

G
genes, 13
genetic mutations, 13

H
HPV vaccine, 43

I
immune system, 26, 30, 41
immunotherapy, 41

J
joints, 4, 31

L
leukemia, 4, 44
lumps, 15

O
oncology, 9
organs, 6, 17, 39

P
prevention, 9, 40, 41, 43
prostate cancer, 18

R
radiation, 17, 26, 28
recurrence, 38, 39
remission, 34, 35, 38, 39
research, 7, 9, 10, 17, 40, 41
researchers, 7, 9, 10, 17, 40, 41
risk factor, 13
risks, 13, 30, 36, 42, 43

S
self-care, 21, 31
side effects, 28, 30, 31, 34, 41
skin cancer, 36
stage of cancer, 15, 20, 21
surgery, 10, 22, 24, 26, 28, 36
survival rates, 32, 40
survivors, 10, 21, 31, 32, 34, 35
symptoms, 15, 18, 34

T
technology, 10
tests, 4, 13, 14, 15, 16, 17, 36, 39
tissue, 17, 22, 39
treatments, 7, 8, 10, 17, 18, 20, 21, 22, 23, 24, 25, 26, 28, 30, 31, 32, 34, 35, 36, 38, 39, 40, 41, 44
tumor, 8, 16, 22, 23, 28
types of cancer, 8, 9, 14, 15, 17, 18, 20, 22, 23, 38, 39, 41, 42, 43

V
vaccines, 43